Nail Fungus & Health Treatment

"Fix Your Fingernail's Health and Look Beautiful"

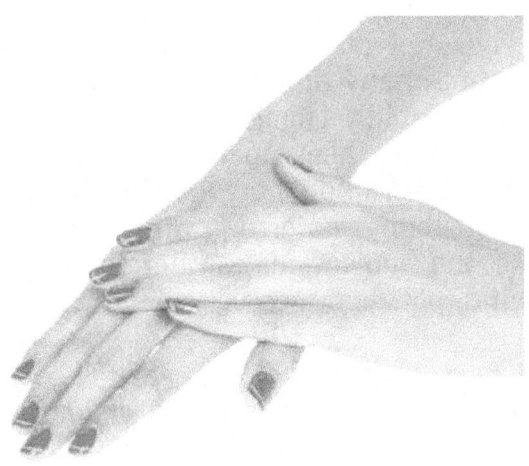

By Rudy S Silva, Natural Nutritionist

Nail Fungus & Health Treatment © 2013 by Rudy S Silva

ISBN-13: 978-1490318813
ISBN-10: 149031881X

Disclaimer and Terms of Use: The Author and Publisher has strived to be as accurate and complete as possible in the creation of this book, notwithstanding the fact that he does not warrant or represent at any time that the contents within are accurate due to the rapidly changing nature of the Internet. While all attempts have been made to verify information provided in this publication, the Author and Publisher assumes no responsibility for errors, omissions, or contrary interpretation of the subject matter herein. Any perceived slights of specific persons, peoples, or organizations are unintentional.

This book intended for use as educational information and if you feel like you need a doctor's opinion, then you should seek it. Use this information for your own education and not as medical advice or treatment. Some of the natural remedies listed here may not have had FDA approval.

All readers are advised to seek services of competent professionals in legal, business, accounting, medical and finance field.

Printed in the United States of America

Table of Contents

1: Introduction – Why You Need Nail Health

Most women and a few men pay a lot of attention to how their fingernails look, but not in terms of their health. It is only when their fingernails become diseased or unsightly that most people get concerned about their fingernails. In this book, your view of fingernails and health, hopeful can change.

Your fingernail condition and their appearance change as you age. When you reach 25 or so, your nail growth rate will slow down. After 35, you may be more susceptible to brittle or splitting nails. By 55, your nails become easily broken and lose their healthy appearance. At any age, you should be concerned about the appearance and health of your nails.

Fingernails may be something you seldom think about, until they start to create pain or look unsightly. Or, if they tend to snag on clothes, fabrics, and cause runs in nylons.

Causes of Fingernail Problems

When fingernails have abnormalities or look unhealthy and don't grow like they should, the cause is often a nutritional imbalance, which comes from a poor diet, eating disorders, digestive issues, or absorption problems.

However, it is possible that nail abnormalities are a reflection of a more serious body condition or disease. Listed here are many different diseases associated with nail appearance.

Many women spend a lot of money on various products to make their nails look better, when their nail appearance starts to diminish. Unfortunately, these products such as nail polish,

polish removers, glues, cements and strengtheners are harsh on fingernail health.

If you are suffering from fingernail or toenail issues, here you will find a number of natural remedies and supplements that will help you strengthen your nails and eliminate fungus or bacteria that have attacked your nails.

If you are a painter, man or a woman, who works with paints, paint thinners, and turpentine, your fingernails are probably in need of help. You will get this help here.

Those of you that work on computers, do manual typing, or play piano have one benefit other might not have. Your continually tapping leads to healthier fingernails.

Included in this book is a diet that gives your overall body the nutrients you need to improve your immune system. Your immune system strength is the key to dealing with fingernail issues and diseases you may have created.

The health of your fingernails is a reflection of your overall health. Nails should be taken care of just like any other part of your body. They should not be used as tools or abused by putting them into harsh liquids.

Even though some people take care of their fingernails, they may still have weak, brittle, peeling, or chipping nails. The actual health of your fingernails is dependent on your overall health.

There are a lot of outside body warnings that your health is below normal and your nails are one of these indicators.

There are two areas that affect the health of your nails and their strength – external and internal. When these areas are not considered, your nails and surrounding skin will not be strong and healthy, which will allow fungus or bacterial to take hold.

External Conditions

There are certain external factors that affect your nails. Fingernails can be damage when placed in strong cleaning solutions that you use to clean your house or scrub floors. If you frequently wash certain clothes by hand with harsh soaps, this will harm your fingernails. Placing your hands in water to wash dishes or other products is damaging to your nails. Also, damaging is the constant heat exposure to your hands.

Aside from fingernail external damage, your cuticles can get torn or ragged. This creates an opening where fungus can get underneath your nails.

Other harsh conditions are frequent gardening or other activities where you use your hands.

Using nail acetone remover, frequently, will make your nails brittle. Nervous conditions where you bite or pick at your nails, will affect the health of your nails and surrounding area.

Internal Conditions

There are many different adverse conditions that can occur on your fingernails or toenails. One of the most common is fungus or bacterial infections that occur under your nails. These are sometimes difficult to cure, since it's hard to get remedies or medication under your nails. Typically, the fungus that develops under your nails is Candida, and it may require antibiotic to eliminate.

Internal Conditions

The degradation of your nail's health can come from kidney, liver, heart, lung, or thyroid disease. It can come from skin diseases like psoriasis or from some hand trauma.

When you see a sudden change in your fingernail's health as revealed in this book, consider this a warning that your health has taken a turn and may warrant a doctor' visit.

In some cases, the materials used in lengthening nails can cause allergic reactions in some women.

If you feel you are in good health, and your nails are brittle and keep breaking, then it may be related to the way you are using your hands. Review your work habits to see if this could be the case. Otherwise, it may be that your health does need improvement. Follow some of the recommendations listed here to improve your health.

2: Fingernail Conditions and Health

Fingernail deteriorating conditions can be reversed by diet and supplements. If you have a fungus or bacterial infection, these can be eliminated using natural antibacterial and fungal remedies.

There are many different fingernail conditions that related to specific deficiency in your body or to the way you polish your nails. Learn these conditions, so that you know what you need to do to regain your health and improve your nail's condition.

Research has found that most of the chipping, brittleness, and weakness of your nails are related to the overuse of nail polishing and nail care products.

It is recommended that you don't use nail strengthening products, since they do more harm than good.

One of the main culprits for nail damage is the adhesive that is used for nails. Acrylic glue resins because a large number of problems, such as cracked, misshapen, thicken, and discolored nails. Permanent disfigurement can occur when using these glues.

Your Nails

Your fingernail is called "nail plate." The fleshy part where your nail plate sits is called the "nail bed. The nail plate grows out of a pale half-moon – lunula - that is at the base of your fingernail. The lunula, which is at the end of the nail and near your skin, contains living cells.

The cuticle serves to attach the skin of your finger to the fingernail. This cuticle is a seal that keeps out dirt, objects, or organisms from getting between your nail plate and nail bed.

It is important not to damage the cuticle.

Under your fingernails are many nerve endings. This is the reason you experience pain, when you have nail fungus or damaged nails.

Your fingernails are made of a protein called keratin and sulfur, which is what hair is made of. Keratin provides your nails with hardness. This keratin grows around 1/8 inch per month and takes 3 months to completely grow out. However, if you lose a fingernail, it will take about 6 to 7 months to completely grow out.

Your nails also need moisture, like your hair, to be smooth and flexible.

A Health Nail

A health nail should appear pink with no spots or discoloration. The nail should be smooth with no ridges, indentations, bumps, pits, or dips.

Unhealthy Nail

Here are some symptoms and appearance of unhealthy nails. Read them over and take notice if you have these conditions. It is these conditions that you need to watch for, as you make changes in your diet, supplements, and washing with harsh chemicals.

- Pale or blue appearance or white or red streaks
- Cracked, brittle or breaking fingernails
- Thick nail, curved and yellow

- Nail separation from bed
- Spoon like nails
- Pitting nails
- White spots on nails
- Nail ridges
- Yellow nails
- Brown nails
- Thickened nails
- Club nails
- Shedding nails
- Horizontal ridges
- Vertical ridges – see anemia deficiency below
- Splitting nails – see low stomach acid.
- hangnails

Pale Or Blue Appearance Or White Or Red Streaks

Nails with pale appearance can occur when you have poor blood circulation.

Cracked, Brittle Or Breaking Fingernails

Cracked nails are usually caused by over use of dish washing soaps or the drying effects of nail polish solvents, like acetone. These effects can be countered by taking a rest from nail polishing and using gloves when washing.

Thick Nails, Curved and Yellow

Curved and yellow nails can be an indication of decreased blood circulation and pulmonary issues. These conditions can be indicators of heart or lung disease.

It is recommended not to have fingernails longer than 1/4 inch past the nail bed. Longer than that tends to interfere with daily activities and become more susceptible to breakage.

Nail Separation from Bed

Nail separation is when the nail plate separates from the nail bed starting at the top of the nail. This can happen when you incur an injury, have an allergic reaction, have poor blood circulation, react to a drug, or react to formaldehyde. Formaldehyde is found most nail hardener that you may be using.

Spoon like Nails

A dip in your nails that takes the shape of a spoon can be an indication of iron deficiency. To verify this, you may need to have some blood tests.

Pitting Nails

Tiny pits that appear on the top of your nail plate can be caused by a fungal infection. In this type of infection, the nail plate will change in color to yellow, brown, or green. For this infection, you will need antibiotics or an antifungal cream.

White Spots On Nails

White spots can be cause by the lack of zinc. However, if you are in good health, there may be no reason for these white spots to appear.

Nail Ridges

If you have ridge-like appearance that occurs from one side of your nail to the other side, this may be caused by a serious illness. When you have a severe illness, nutrients do not reach your nails or hair. The result is that you have fingernails that look jagged all along the edges.

Yellow Nails

Yellow nails reflect an illness in your circulatory system. Yellow nails may also appear as you age, which indicate a need for more nutritional food.

Brown Nails

A greenish, brown nail appearance can be an indication of a fungal infection. This infection is under the nail plate and can be hard to treat.

Thickened Nails

Thickened nails can occur when you have an allergic reaction to formaldehyde. It is also be caused by a fungal infection.

Club Nails

Club nails appear round and are a sign of lung and/or heart disease. When you improve these issues your nails can return to normal.

Shedding Nails

This condition is where the tips of your nails are ragged and chipped. This occurs as a result of an injury or fungal infection.

Horizontal Ridges

Horizontal ridges can be a sign of a nutritionally poor diet.

This type of sign is typically associated with those that go on a crash diet and don't eat nutritional food. However, there are many people who do not have a good diet and become deficient in many different nutrients. This creates many different diseases that are reflected in the health of their nails.

Hangnails

Hangnails occur from a lack of protein, folic acid, and vitamin C. White bands across your nails also indicate a lack of protein.

Other Disorders Visible In Nails

Here are some addition signs and conditions of unhealthy nail and body conditions.

- Black, splinter like bits under your nails - this can be a sign of heart infections

- Black bands starting from the cuticle to tips of your nails – this can be a sign of melanoma

- Crumbly, white nails near the cuticle – this can be a sign of AIDS

- Deep-blue nail beds or nails that cure downward– indicate asthma or emphysema

- Flat nails – can indicate Raynaud's disease

- Nails that have the top half white and the other half pink – indicates kidney problems

- Chipping, peeling, cracking, thinning, and breaking nails – indicate a nutritional problem

- Thick nails – indicate a thyroid problem or poor blood circulation

- White lines across the nail – may indicate a liver disease

Using Your Hands

Whenever you are washing with harsh chemicals, without gloves, you are exposing your fingernails to harm. When you wash and your nails get wet, they swell and when you dry them, they shrink. Over time your nails will become brittle and delicate.

If you live in cold weather or dry heated rooms, your nails over time can also become brittle or develop other problems.

Use gloves for your washing projects when possible. When finished with your work, wash your hands, dry, and then put a moisturizing cream on your hands and fingernails.

You can also get into the habit of carrying around a cream for your fingernails and using it when you are not busy, during the day. Over time you will see improvement in your nail health.

Nail Polish

Acetone Nail polish remover has the power to dry your nails and can harm them over long term use. Try to use a polish remover that contains acetates. Cutting into your cuticles during manicures can cause damage to the nail. The cuticle provides protection for your nail bed against damage and infection.

Brittle Nails

If you are using gloves and creams on your hands and nails

and see no improvement in 3 months, then you may have a nutritional deficiency or some other disease.

Thyroid Function

If you have poor nails, thin hair, and lack energy, this could be from a poor functioning thyroid, since your thyroid controls burning of food for your body's energy. A low thyroid function can affect the amount of nutrients your nails get.

Low Stomach Acid

Splitting nails is one symptom of low stomach acid. In addition, poor digestion and absorption can prevent you from getting the nutrients you need for good nail health. Low stomach acid can cause cracked, peeling or weak nails. Weak stomach acid comes from a poor diet or from frequent use of drugstore medication for acid reflux or heartburn. The diet discussed here will help you improve your stomach acid levels.

In his book, Why Stomach Acid Is Good for You, Jonathan V. Wright, M.D. and Lane Lenard, Ph.D., say that,

"In a way, women with low stomach acid are often 'lucky' to develop one of two 'signs' that men with the same problem rarely encounter: cracking, chipping, peeling, and 'layering' fingernails, or overall (not localized) head hair loss (it's rare to have both poor-quality fingernails and hair loss occur in the same woman.)

...women with these problems know something's the matter and sometimes are also lucky enough to find nutritionally oriented physicians who will help these symptoms to diagnose and correct or compensate for the underlying cause: poor stomach function. 'Patching up' the stomach problem helps not only the hair loss and the 'lousy' fingernails, but the entire body's nutrition as well!"

Iron Deficiency Anemia

If you are anemic, expect to have brittle, spoon shaped, indentations, vertical ridges, or dips in your nails. Iron is necessary for healthy nails. It is always safe to get your iron with a doctor's prescription. If you are anemic then check out this **Anemia Kindle** to see how you can fight anemia using natural foods and remedies.

Now, you can see that your fingernails are not just for decoration. They are indicators of your health. Covering up their poor appearance with polish, delays the health issue you need to deal with. Take some time to examine your nails and decide what action you need to take after reading the rest of this book.

Care For Nails

When you trim your nails, don't round your nails. Leave them square at the corner, if you have weak nails.

Always be prepared to file off nicks or chips that appear on your nails. This keeps you from further nail damage.

Use nail remover only once a week or longer. Look for alternatives to acetone nail polish remover. Acetone will dry your nails and is toxic. It is easily absorbed into your blood.

Artificial Fingernails

Avoid using artificial fingernails over your nails. They destroy your nails. The chemicals and glue you need to use are dangerous and toxic to your body. The chemicals will crack your nail plate and damage your nail bed. This is one reason why these artificial nails often lead to a fungus infection.

Manicures

If you have manicures, make sure they clean their instruments with isopropyl alcohol. You can always bring your own tools to have a manicure.

3: Getting Rid Of Toxins for Nail Health

One of the first things you need to do to get started on getting healthier nails is to do a two to three-day colon and blood cleanse. You might think this is a lot of work to do cleanse, but this is a quick and easy one. Besides you need to do some house cleaning in your body to make this program more effective.

This is an important step, because you want to remove toxins and mucus from your intestinal tract – stomach, small intestine, colon, and many other body organs. In this three day cleanse, you will also remove toxins from within your cells and lymph liquid.

Pulling Out Acids and Toxins

This cleanse will pull out many acids, acid wastes, and toxins you have floating around in your body. This is particularly important, if you have a fungus or bacterial infection. Also, removing excess acids from your body moves your body toward an alkaline state, and this is the condition where you harbor less disease.

This cleanse will clean out your blood and neutralize many of the acids in your body that are causing you harm. The cleanse will also pull out excess body water and reduce any edema that you might have. This will happen because this cleanse promotes urination and bowel movements.

This will improve your immune system and give you better nail health.

So, here's what you need to do to get started.

The Day Before The Cleanse

Buy the following juices for this cleanse a few days before or the day before your cleanse.

- Organic apple juice – one gallon
- Organic apples – 3 for one day, 10 apples for three days
- Organic prune juice – 1/2 gallon
- Organic Cherry juice – 1/2 gallon
- Carrots for your juicer or carrot juice – one quart

The day before the fast, eat a large salad and two apples at dinner time. This will give you plenty of fiber to scrub the walls of your colon as you move fecal matter out of your colon the following day.

Cleansing The Colon

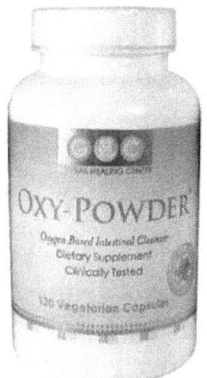

If you chose to use Oxy-Powder, then here is where you can buy it on the Internet: Get Oxy-Powder

The night before you start your weight loss program, take four Oxy-Powder capsules. If you need to lose a lot of weight, then take five capsules the night before and just before you go to bed.

Now, Oxy-Powder is not a laxative so they are not addictive. What these capsules do is supply oxygen to your colon, which dissolves the hard fecal matter that has built up over time and has not wanted to come out.

Because this bottle of Oxy-Powder has 125 capsules, you can

take 1 to 3 capsules during your 10 day weight loss program.

Oxy-Powder causes your stools to become watery, since it is dissolving the hard matter in your colon. Don't be concern that you have diarrhea like symptoms. Also this three day cleanse will also cause you to have watery stools, since you are on a diet of juices and Gouts.

If you chose to use prune juice to clear out your colon, this procedure will be described below.

First day of colon cleanse

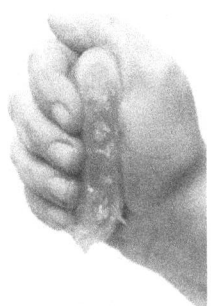

Do this cleanse on a Saturday, Sunday or any other day that you don't have to go anywhere. You may be going to the bathroom all day and at times you need to be there quick. But, you can do this cleanse even during a work day.

This first morning, you will have a bowel movement when you wake up, because of the Oxy-Powder. After that, go do your lemon drink.

Lemon Juice Drink - Every morning when you first get up, drink a glass of slightly warm water with the juice of 1/2 lemon. This will remove mucus from your intestinal tract and detoxify your liver.

Prune Juice Colon Cleanse

If you decided to use prune juice to clean out your colon, instead of Oxy-Powder, then here is what you need to do.

But, you can also do prune juice, if you have done the Oxy-powder, since the prune juice is filled with minerals and nutrients that will help cleanse your body more.

- About 1/2 hour after your lemon drink, take 8 oz. of prune juice.
- 10 minutes later drink another 8 oz. of prune juice
- 10 minutes later again drink another 8 oz. of prune juice
- 20 minutes than drink 8 oz. of apple juice
- 30 minutes than drink another 8 oz. of apple juice

If you haven't sped to the bathroom yet, you will in a little while.

Now drink 8 oz. of apple juice every hour until the end of the day. You can stop drinking apple juice around 5pm. You can use different fruit juices or vegetable juices in place of apple juice, but, just make sure you drink mostly apple juice.

During the day you can eat 1 or 2 apple in the morning and 1 in the evening.

Second Day Of The Colon Cleanse

During the second day, you can drink different kinds of juices and eat 2-6 apples. You can drink any kind of juice be it fruit or vegetable. A combination of fruit and vegetable juice is good. You can also eat other fruits, such as watermelon, melon, oranges, and strawberries.

Third Day Of The Colon Cleanse

The third day is like the second day, where you can drink different kinds of juice and eat 2-6 apples or other fruits.

On this day you can eat other fruits like mango, watermelon, cantaloupe, and pineapple. At the end of this day, you can eat a salad with a variety of vegetables.

Fourth Day Start Of Colon Cleanse

You can continue to use Oxy-powder at 2 capsules every night for the rest of the month.

4: Minerals In Fruits Give You Fantastic Nails

Minerals

Moving your body more toward alkalinity is what will give you the best health. When you have fingernail problems, getting more minerals in your body is the first step. An alkaline body prevents your body from becoming ill and forming deadly diseases, like joint problems, organ degradation, body pain, skin eruptions, cancer, and system weaknesses.

If you are already sick, then all of the chemicals inside fruits and vegetables will help revive you to better health. This is provided that your tissue damage has not gone beyond repair. Having illness is not good for your nails, since they will not receive the nutrients they need to prevent them from being unsightly.

The minerals most important in changing and maintaining your body in an alkaline condition are sodium, potassium, chloride, calcium, phosphorus, magnesium, and sulfur.

Acid Binding

There are certain minerals that are called acid binding. These are the minerals mentioned earlier and are the most important ones in fruits - sodium, potassium, chloride, calcium, phosphorus, magnesium.

What acid binding means is when you eat fruits with these minerals, your cells, after metabolism, create an alkaline ash. This ash will seek out acids in your body and bind with them to neutralize them. These captured acids are now routed out of your body through your urine, stools, and breathe.

So you can see the importance of getting a lot of alkaline minerals into your body. Without them, acids which do not get bonded to alkaline minerals would move back into your body tissue and continue their body damage.

Body Detoxification

The highest priority of the body is to detoxify itself. One of the best way to help your body detoxify is to provide minerals that bind with acids that are in the cells, tissues, organs, and muscles. What these alkaline acid binding minerals do is to pull out the toxins that are dispersed throughout your body.

Body Organs

All body organs function to rid the body of acid waste or toxins. Lack of acid binding food causes deterioration of the function of these organs. Each organ has a specific function in the elimination and neutralization of acid wastes and it does this in conjunction with acid binding minerals.

The Acid Binding Fruits To Eat

Here is a list of fruits, vegetables that have the highest alkaline minerals. The percentage number next to these foods indicates the strength of the alkaline minerals or the acid binding power.

The closer to 100% the more effective these foods are as an acid reducing food. However you should be eating all foods throughout the list not just the ones at the top of the list.

The percentage assigned to these fruits and vegetables is based on fresh fruits and vegetables that are organic and not cooked, canned or mixed with sugar. If they are cook or otherwise processed in some fashion, this will slightly reduce their effectiveness as an acid binding. However, they will still be effective in acid binding.

Here is the list of foods to eat in the order of priority.

Fruits

1. Fruits at 100% Acid Binding – Best Fruits To Eat Lemons, melons – any type, watermelon

2. Fruits at 93% Acid Binding – Great Fruits To Eat Cantaloupes, dried dates, dried figs, limes, mango, papaya

3. Fruits at 87% Acid Binding – Still Great Fruits To Eat Kiwis, passion fruit, pineapples, raisins, umeboshi plums

4. Fruits at 80% Acid Binding – Eat These Fruits Apricots, avocados, bananas, fresh dates, fresh figs, currants, gooseberries grapes, grapefruits guavas, kumquats, nectarines, pears, persimmons, quince, berries, cactus

5. Fruits at 73% Acid Binding – Still Fruits To Eat Apples, oranges, peaches, pomegranate, raspberries, sour grapes, strawberries, carob

6. Fruits at 67% Acid Binding – Still Neutralizes Acids Cherries, fresh coconut

7. Herbal Teas From Leaves at 73% to 86% acid binding Alfalfa, mint, sage, spearmint, raspberry strawberry comfrey

8. All fruit Juices from a juicer 100% Acid Binding

Vegetables

Here is the list of vegetables to eat in order of priority. All of these vegetables will neutralize acid, since they contain minerals that are acid binding.

1. Vegetables at 93% Acid Binding – best vegetables to eat
   Kelp, **Seaweed**, Watercress, Asparagus

2. Vegetables at 80% Acid Binding – Still the best to eat
   Lettuce Leaf, Oyster plant, Pumpkin, Spinach, **Collard greens** Squash, Peas, **Carrots, Celery**, Chard, Swiss, Dandelion greens

3. Vegetables at 73% Acid Binding – Great vegetables to eat
   Bamboo shoots, Beets, **Broccoli**, Cabbage, Cauliflower, Collards, Corn, sweet, Ginger (fresh), Mushrooms, Mustard greens, Onions, Pepper, Potatoes, Green, Lima, String, Potatoes

4. Vegetables at 67% Acid Binding – eat plenty of these
   Brussels sprouts, **Cucumbers**, Eggplant, Okra, Onions, Radishes, Tomatoes

5. Vegetable juices at 80% to 93% Acid Binding
   Parsley, wheat grass, carrot, celery, etc.

5: How to Eat For Nail Health

Here is the way you should be eating breakfast and fruits. By using this process, you will start to move your body to a more alkaline state. This is the state you want to achieve in your body, because this is the condition where you have fewer illnesses.

If you don't improve your health, it will be difficult to maintain good fingernail and toenail health. You will be constantly dealing with poor fingernail conditions and fungus, especially if you are always painting your nails and getting pedicures and manicures.

If you have other illnesses that are causing your nails to appear unsightly, then eating your breakfast as recommended here will help you to eliminate some of these body conditions.

Body Cycles

Body cycles are time periods where your body is doing certain functions in your body. It does this automatically as if it was on a timer. Knowing what these functions are will help you get relief from your nail disease.

In this book, we discuss only the first body cycle, since this period is the detoxification time.

Here are the 3 natural body cycles:

Cycle 1 time period: 4 am. to noon

This cycle is the time where your body is eliminating toxins, acids, wastes, and derby through urine, bowel movements, and other secretions. Most people interfere with this cycle, since they are unaware of it, causing constipation, increase weight and various detrimental illnesses.

Cycle 2 time period: noon to 8 pm

This is the time when your body should be taking in food and digesting it. By eating the right kind of food, you help your digestive process in your stomach and small intestine. This is your first and second meal of the day – lunch and dinner.

Cycle 3 time period: 8 pm to 4 am.

This is the time your body is absorbing and using food you have eaten from noon to 8 pm. Various organs are detoxifying and producing waste and moving it into your kidney and colon. When you wake up, this is the waste you should be getting rid during body cycle one.

The First Body Cycle

During the elimination cycle, 4 am. to noon, eat and drink only fruits and their juices or drink vegetable juices. For breakfast, eat a bowl of fruit or have a fruit smoothie made with apple juice, banana, and fruits in season.

Before noontime, eat fruit as snacks. Forty-five minutes before noon eat your last fruit. You can eat and drink all the fruit and juices you want up to noontime.
Fruits contain the right balance of nutrients with about 70% distilled water. Eat them without cooking them. They are easy to digest and absorb and do not stress your colon. They activate peristaltic action in your colon and help you have a bowel movement.

Here are some Acid Binding fruits to eat:

- Apples
- Apricots
- Avocados
- Bananas
- Blueberries
- Boysenberries
- Cantaloupes
- Cherries
- Figs and dates
- Grapes
- Grapes
- Lemons
- Nectarines
- Oranges
- Papayas
- Peaches
- Pears
- Persimmons
- Plums
- Prunes
- Raspberries
- Strawberries
- Watermelons

Eat all melons together and wait 1/2 hour before eating other fruits. Melons require specific enzymes to be digested in the stomach, so other fruit eaten with melons will just sit in your stomach, waiting to be digested and can cause gas or an acid stomach.

By eating fruits during body cycle 1 you are assisting your body's elimination cycle. Fruits and juices help your body to urinate, or have a bowel movement, and eliminate toxins and acids from your body and blood. It is these toxins and acids that make you, overweight, constipated, and sick.

Eating solid food for breakfast – eggs potatoes, rice, meat, cereal, milk, and so on, the typical breakfast, interferes with your body's elimination cycle and eventually leads to sickness and excess weight.

It takes over 3 hours to digest heavy and solid food. The food you should be eating in the morning should digest quickly. This helps you to activate peristaltic colon action to create a bowel movement and to continue your body's detoxification and elimination process.

Heavy food slows down the elimination of toxins from your body, and this causes chime and toxins to remain in your colon longer than necessary. These toxins then get stored in your body as fat and acids.

It takes 1 to 1 1/2 hour or so to digest juices. Because of this, they help to cleanse your body of waste during the time from 4am to noontime.

So if you are not already having fruit and fruit and vegetable juices for breakfast and snacks, start slowing changing your eating habits, if you want to lose weight and feel better.

6: Foods That Bring Nails Back To Health

Protein For Strong Nails

Protein is an essential food for having good nail health. It is the building block of your nails, since it provides keratin. Without the proper amount, you will not be able to absorb the calcium you need in your nails.

Your nails need plenty of protein to maintain a strong and resilient structure. Here is what you need to eat for protein.

- Fish
- Chicken
- Beef
- Beans
- Gelatin deserts
- Crips fresh dark green salads
- Low calorie dairy products
- Whey protein
- Whole grains – brown rice

Biotin Foods

Foods that have biotin are soybeans flour, cauliflower, lentils, and skim or low-fat milk.

Parsnips

Parsnips are not favored by many people because of their taste. Its benefit comes from have all the minerals that are good for an alkaline body. In addition, it has been found to be beneficial for healthy nails, skin, and hair. Here's how to use it.

Juice parsnips and mix it with carrot juice. Work with the mixture you can drink and slowly combine more parsnip juice than carrot. Drink this once a day with your meals.

Silicon

Silicon is necessary for strong nails. Here are a few symptoms of low silicon that you can use to help you identify lack silicon.

- Nervous stomach
- Low body temperature
- Foot perspiration
- Skin disorders
- Fatigue
- Depression
- Slow healing
- Sexual weakness

These are the foods you want to eat for silicon. Even if you don't have these low silicon symptoms, add these foods to your diet. They will help reinforce your nail strength.

- Oats
- Barley
- Nuts, seeds
- Rice bran
- Kelp
- Grains, cereals
- Oat straw tea
- Alfalfa tablets

- Apples, apricots, bananas
- Cabbage
- Raisin
- Brown rice
- Eggs

Food For Your Diet

Here are some of the more important foods to include in your diet for healthy nails.

Fruits and raw vegetables should be 50% of your diet. Use the fruits listed that make your body more alkaline. Also, eat plenty of broccoli, onions, fish, sea vegetables, whole grains

Sea Vegetables

Sea vegetables aid in the growth of nails, hair, bone, and teeth. They aid in the functioning of endocrine glands, especially the thyroid. Here is a list of some of the sea vegetables you can find in your health-food store. Use them in soups and other food preparations.

Kelp, dulse, kombu, kuzu, nori, sea palm, wild nori, wakame, hijiki

Agar Agar

Agar agar can be used in place of gelatin. Gelatin is made from animal protein, whereas, Agar Agar is derived from seaweed. Use this like gelatin. You can make a jello like desert with agar agar. Simply boil water and dissolve it. Then pour it into cups and add honey and other fruits. Let it sit on your table and soon it will gel.

7: Remedies to Eliminate Fungus Nails

Fungus under your nails can result in pain, swelling, and pus. These nails can become white, yellow, and discolored and eventually fall off your fingers.

Keep in mind that not all medications or remedies will work to clear nail infections. For this reason, many different remedies are listed here that you can try for your condition. Whenever you see the first signs of an unwanted nail condition, start right away using the various remedies listed in this book.

When you have fungus, you will have to attack it by using external and internal medication. It may be necessary to get medical help, if you can't eliminate this fungus using natural remedies.

Fungus Remedies and Medication

Getting medication under your nails is one of the challenges in curing infected nails. One effective way to deal with this is by using an antifungal agent ketoconazole that is mixed with dimethylsulfoxide, DMSO. DMSO is known as a carrier and can move a medication or substance from outside the skin deep into the skin where the medication can do its work.

For more information, head over to this website for the **DMSO information**.

Apple cider or Vinegar Treatment

Water
Vitamin E

Mix apple cider vinegar with 1/2 warm water. Place your fingernails or toe nails into this solution for 30 minutes.

Slightly increase the strength of this solution every day, by using more vinegar than water. Dry your nails and rub in the following mixture.

Mix 1/2 vitamin E and 1/2 tree tea oil. Rub this mixture onto your nails. Cut up a vitamin E gel capsule to get the vitamin E your need. You can also use an oregano extract, since it has antibacterial and antifungal properties.

Do this two times a day for two weeks. After you see some improvement or the condition clears, continue using this mixture for one week more.

After Apple Cider Treatment

Here is an additional treatment you can do at the end of the apple cider treatment.

In bowl place 2 tablespoons of backing soda. Now add 1 tablespoon of apple cider vinegar. Create a paste with a good consistency. Rub this mixture onto your infected nail for 30 minutes or so. Do this twice a day.

Vicks Vapor Rub

Using Vicks Vapor Rub is a time tested remedy for clearing up fungus infections. At the first signs of an infection, here's what to do.

Put Vicks all over the infected area and let it air dry.

Do this morning and night. If you work during the day, you may want to put a band aid over the Vicks.

8: Natural Remedies for Stronger and Healthier Nails

Here are some natural remedies that you can make and use to give your nails and cuticles oils and other nutrients.

Oil For Cuticles and Nails

These oils will prevent the formation of hang nails and treat your brittle nails.

- ¼ tsp jojoba oil

- ½ tsp. almond oil

- Vitamin E 400 IU

- 2 drops carrot seed essential oil

- 1 drop eucalyptus essential oil

- 2 drops of lemon essential oil

Now, mix all of these ingredients and place them into a dark dropper bottle, then rub them into your cuticles and nails at least twice a day.

Yes, these are a lot of oil but make a batch and it will last a long time and you can share some with family or friends.
Here is another easier oil mixture to make.

- ¼ tsp. avocado oil

- 20 drops evening primrose oil

- 5 drops grapefruit essential oil

- 5 drops carrot seed essential oil

If you have evening primrose capsules, break them open to get your 20 drops. Mix all of these oils into a dark dropper bottle and apply the oils three times a day.

Yellow Nails

Here's what you can do if you have yellow nails that are brittle and lack texture.

Mix equal parts of honey, avocado oil, and egg yolk with a pinch of salt. Rub this combination into your nails and cuticles and leave it on for 30 minutes every day. You should see results in about two weeks.

Carrot and Cucumber Juice

Cucumber juice mixed with carrot juice provides a high level of silicon and sulfur. This will produce strong nails and prevent them from splitting. This drink contains sodium, potassium, calcium, chlorine, and phosphorus, all which contribute to make your body more alkaline.

Parsnip Juice

Parsnip juice has a high level of silicon and sulfur, which is beneficial for brittle nails. If you would like to try this juice, mix it with carrot juice to make it more palatable. In all juices that you make, you can add some apple juice to improve the taste.

Soaking In Water

In their book, High Speed Healing, by the Editors of Prevention Magazine Health Books, 1991, they recommend the following.

"Your brittle nails will benefit most from a nightly soak in plain warm water. Fifteen to 20 minutes of soaking is best, says Richard K Scher, M.D. from the Columbia Presbyterian Medical Center in New York. If you have a favorite before-bed television program, you can soak your nails and watch at the same time. Once 20 minutes have elapsed, dry your nails and apply a moisturizer."

If your nails are brittle, you can also soak them in water and bath oil 10 to 15 minutes, then clip them.

Epilyt and Elon

Here are two products you might want to try on your nails. Epilyt is made for rough and scaly skin. Some people have found this product also good for nail health.

Elon is a product especially made for nails. It is antifungal and contains other ingredients to help penetrate your nails. Using this product should show results for weak nails in 3 to 4 weeks.

Horse Remedy

In their book, The People's Pharmacy Guide to Home and Herbal Remedies, Joe Graedon and Teresa Graedon, PhD, tell about a horse remedy,

"Ten years ago, the owners of a feed and garden store in Texas alerted us to the fact that a lot of their female customers were buying hoot moisturizers. The horse women in their area discovered that when they used their hands to apply such products to their horse's hooves, their own fingernails seemed harder and stronger. The word has gotten out because the owners confided: 'About 80 percent of our sales are to women who don't usually shop in a feed store. We sell both **Purina Hoof Moisturizer** and **Hoofmaker** ...'"

This moisturizer contains lanolin, beeswax, mineral oil, and coconut oil.

You can also use **T-Hoof Equine Hoof Moisturizer** and Conditioner.

Here is a testimonial for this product.

"T-Hoof Equine Hoof Moisturizer and Conditioner Best Stuff Ever BY: 1percheron (LEDYARD, CT) - Jan 24, 2013   ITEM #: 34092

T-Hoof is The Best Stuff Ever. Really! It absorbs quickly and conditions instantly, is not greasy or oily, doesn't attract dirt, dust, or barn detritus. It actually allows me to keep my horse barefoot, even in the dry weather of summer! And, as a plus, it's awesome for my hands and fingernails. My fingernails have never been so strong, and they seem to grow quicker! I love this stuff. I keep a jar of it at my desk at work and co-workers always stop by for some."

Horsetail Herb

Horsetail herb has a history, throughout Europe and China, of providing nutrients for maintaining strong nails. It is high in silica or silicon. Its nutrients facilitate the absorption of calcium, which nourishes nails, skin, bones, and hair.

Horsetail herb is a good nail conditioner and helps to eliminate white spots on your nails, which may be a sign zinc deficiency.

Almond or Olive Oil Treatment

For dry, brittle, splitting nails and ragged cuticles use a hot almond or olive oil treatment. In a bowl, put some warm almond or olive oil and soak your fingernail tips into the oil for 10 to 15 minutes.

You can also place your nails into apple cider vinegar for 10 minutes every day, to strengthen your nails.

Bed Time

Just before going to bed, coat your hands and nails with petroleum jelly. Then put some cotton gloves and leave them on overnight. This will keep your nails moist and prevent them from becoming brittle.

Herbs to Strengthen Nails

Here is a combination of herbs in capsule form to feed your fingernails.

- Dulse

- Horsetail

- Sage

- Rosemary

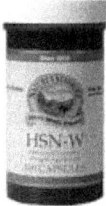

Here is where you can find this combination on the internet – **HSN-W**.

What this herbal formula, HSN-W, does is provide your body with a high amount of silica. Silica is one of the important ingredients that will improve the health of your fingernails.

Because this product also contains other minerals like iron, zinc, magnesium, and chromium, it enhances the formation and structure of your nails.

Knox Gelatin

Knox is known as a remedy for weak and brittle nails. You can mix one packet with water and drink it each day. It will provide you with plenty of protein for your nails.

Chaparral Herbal Tea

Chaparral is an excellent blood purifier and is useful for removing toxins from your blood and lymph liquid. For nail fungus conditions, prepare a tea and drink it every day. You can buy this herb at herbal shops and prepare a tea as follows. Boil distilled water and add a tablespoon of chaparral herb. Turn fire off and let solution sit for 10 to 15 minutes. Drink a cup of this tea every day for 21 days. You may want to add some honey if it's too bitter for you.

In addition, you can put your infected fingers or toes into this tea for 15 minutes each day.

Garlic Application

Garlic is also an antifungal herb. You can buy garlic oil and apply it directly onto your infected area. When you use this method, you should also take garlic powdered capsules to attack this fungus internally.

Brewer's Yeast

For splitting nails or hangnails use two tablespoons of brewer's yeast to get the B vitamins and many minerals your nails need.

Natural Nail Polish

Here is a more natural nail polish you can use that doesn't have harsh chemicals.

Drs Remedy Rescue Nail Polish

This nail polish promotes nail health, since it does not have the harsh commercial chemicals that many other nail polishs have. It also contains antifungal chemicals to keep your nails healthy.

9: Supplements for Superior Nail Health

Using supplements is a necessary step to add force to your immune system. Supplements help you rebuild the health of your entire body, during a time that you need additional nutrition. After you experience some nail health recovery, you can back off on supplements and depend on a good diet to provide you with the nutrition your body needs.

Vitamin A

Add vitamin A to your diet. Your will not be able to absorb the protein you eat, without adequate vitamin A. This vitamin helps to prevent nail dryness and brittleness. Use it in conjunction with calcium.

Use up to 25,000 IU except if you are pregnant, and then only use up to 10,000 IU.

Vitamin C

Your body uses a tremendous amount of vitamin C. Most people are always short on this vitamin. Vitamin C is necessary for a strong immune system. Without a strong immune system, it will be difficult for you to get rid of any fungus that attacks your nails.

Use 3000 to 4000 mg of vitamin C per day.

Calcium

Because your nails contain calcium, you will need to take a calcium supplement. Take a minimum of 1500 mg per day.

When taking calcium always use a supplement that contains magnesium and vitamin D to absorb more calcium.

Use Calcium Citrate

Biotin

Biotin is an important mineral needed for nail health. It helps to improve nail hardness, firmness, and thickness. Studies have shown that by using up to 2,500ug of biotin a day, you can increase your nail thickness by 25 percent. This amount of biotin is more than you need. The Daily Value recommends 300ug per day but you can take double this amount, when you have nail issues.

You can take a vitamin B complex, such as the B100 to satisfy your vitamin B requirements.

The lack of vitamin B causes horizontal and vertical lines in your nails.

Iron

With your doctor's care, take iron if you have anemia.

Probiotic

A supplement of friendly bacteria is necessary to improve your digestion and to provide bacteria that fight fungus that gets under your fingernails. Use one capsule per day between meals.

MSM

If you want hard nails, MSM is necessary for good hard fingernails. Your nails need keratin and they can get it from MSM. MSM contains 30% sulfur and one of the amino acids that you need, which is made from sulfur – cystine. Cystine is one of the building blocks of keratin. Not only is MSM fantastic for nails, it will provide you with nutrients for keeping your hands soft and your hair and completion beautiful.

Take 2000 to 4000 mg MSM per day.

Take this for 3 months for the best results. Go here to get the **best MSM** in 1000 mg torpedoes, which are easy to swallow.

MSM is also good for constipation and when you take a lot of MSM your bowel movements may become more frequent. However, this might occur when you take 6000 to 10,000 mg. Having more bowel movements, 2-3 per day, is typically good for your health.

Fish Oil

Fish oil is always a necessity for any type of body issue that you are trying to correct. Dry nails can benefit by the consistent use of fish oil or any of the other essential oils. Eating fish is also beneficial for getting the protein and the omega-3 and 6.

Silicon

Silicon is used throughout your body for bone, skin, artery, and nail strength. Since this is a trace mineral, you only need a small amount, like 10 to 20 mg per day.

Zinc

A deficiency of zinc leads to weak nails. Here is the dose to take.
Use 30 mg of zinc per day.

L-Methionine

If you eat little meat or are a vegetarian, you need to

supplement with L-Methionine, an antioxidant. This amino acid is necessary to strengthen nails.

Use 1500 mg per day of L-Methionine

10: How to Fix Your Nail Problems

Now, you have plenty of information to define a diet which is supported by remedies and supplements. With all this information, it can be difficult to determine where to start. Here is an outline that you can start with. You can vary this program, since you have a variety of different nutrients and remedies to use.

You should not try to use all of them, but try to pick one or two to start with to see what your response is. If you do not get any results with a specific remedy, move on to another remedy. Look at the foods you should be eating and add them to your typical diet.

Here's a program to get your started.

1. Start out with at least a two-day body cleanse. You want to get your body thinking about releasing toxins and this is an excellent way to do it.

2. If you have fingernail fungus, then pick a remedy and apply it for at least one week. By that time, you should be able to tell if it's going to work. If it works, then continue using it for another week.

3. Look at the body cycles and start following cycle one, where you only eat fruits and vegetable juices from morning to noon. Eat those fruits that will give you the maximum benefit for an alkaline body to start with.

4. It's important to eat only fruits in the morning to continue to detoxify and de-acidify your body. This will

strengthen your immune and digestive system. You need a strong digestive system to digest and absorb nutrients from the food you eat.

5. Look at the foods you need to eat to strengthening your nails. Incorporate those foods into your diet. Eat oats, nuts, seeds, broccoli, onions, garlic, cabbage, protein, agar agar, sea vegetables and so on. Make a list of the foods you want to buy at the store.

6. Look at the natural remedies that will strengthen your nails for specific conditions and chose one to use, for example, herbal formula HSN-W.

7. Look at the supplements and try to find a complex that contains many of the vitamins and minerals listed. Sometimes, you can find a supplement that is for **strong nails**. Be sure to include an MSM supplement.

8. Take care of your hands using gloves when necessary. Sometimes its extra work to use gloves, but it's worth it over the long term.

11: Author and Resources

Get one of my best kindle books *free* below:

http://www.natural-remedies-thatwork.com

Rudy Silva is a natural nutritional consultant educated in the United States in Nutrition and Physics. He is a graduate from San Jose State University in California. He is author of 45 other books on natural remedies. He has authored a newsletter in natural remedies for over 10 years.

Resource page

Here are some of the other kindle e-books about natural remedies that have been written by this author. You can see the entire list at:

http://tinyurl.com/b2f7wd3

Acne Remedies
- Best natural acne treatments: Acne facial
- Effective Acne Treatments That Work

Constipation Remedies
- The Best Constipation Remedies
- Best Constipated Women Natural Cures
- How To Relieve Constipation With Fruits

Essential Fatty Acids
- Taking The Mystery Out Of Essential Fatty acids
- Amazing Fish Oil Benefits Revealed
- Omega 3 and 6 Mystery Exposed

Nutrition Remedies
- Updated Version - Secret Diet And Nutrition

- Fantastic Alkaline Fruit Benefits Revealed
- Calcium (Discover How To Use Calcium To Avoid Devastating Diseases)
- Magnesium Nutrition Revealed
- Best Nutrition Health Practices
- Potassium Health Secrets Revealed
- Phosphorus, The Best Brain Food
- A Sodium Diet (What You Must Know About Sodium)

Stomach Remedies
- Acid Reflux: Fast and Easy Cures For Acid Reflux
- Asthma Treatment Cures With Remedies
- How To Do Natural Colon Cleansing

Misc Remedies
- Natural Hair Loss Treatment: Women And Men
- Effective Natural Hemorrhoids Treatment
- Iron Deficiency Anemia
- Secrets To Understanding Behavior
- Fast Acting Ear Infection Remedies
- What Is A Hiatus Hernia
- Best Varicose Vein Treatments?
- Make Shampoos At Home Using Natural
- Ingredients:Discover recipes for quality natural hair shampoos
- How To Fix Your Thyroid Problems: Discover Hidden Ideas That Fix Your Thyroid
- Nail Fungus & Health Treatment: Fix Your Fingernail's Health And Look Beautiful
- Diarrhea: How To Stop Diarrhea Chronic Or Severe

Minerals
- Calcium and Magnesium Magic Body Benefits Revealed
- The Magic of Sodium, Calcium and Magnesium
- Create an Alkaline Body with Potassium and Sodium: Eliminate a Potassium Deficiency

- Calcium and Phosphorus Foods: Deficiency or Excesses in These Minerals Cause Bone and Brain Power Loss

Men's Health
- Best Impotence Health Diet

Weight loss
- Ten (10) Day Quick Success Weight Loss Program: A new approach to losing weight by changing your eating habits for life
- Discover Secret Anti-Aging Juice & Tonic Recipes: Unique Juices And Tonics That Create Beauty And Youth

To see all the kindle books written by this author, go to this the Authors Profile Page or this URL,

http://tinyurl.com/b2f7wd3

If you need support or want to promote any of his e-books, please contact him at rss41@yahoo.com and expect a reply within 24 hours. He looks forward to hearing from you and is happy to help you understand his material on natural and nutritional health.

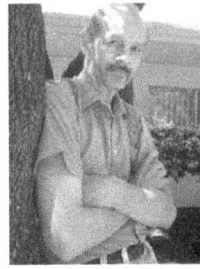

Give A Review

And, don't for get to give a review for this e-book at Amazon so that others can gain the benefits of what is in this e-book. To you, for losing weight, creating better health and more happiness in your life,

Rudy S Silva